VEGAN FIRST STEPS
A quick-start guide to healthy veganism

by Rachel Iris Jimenez

ISBN-13: 978-1497435131

ISBN-10: 1497435137

www.veganfirststeps.com

TABLE OF CONTENTS

INTRODUCTION

I am not a doctor or nutritionist. I am just someone who over the years has undergone a transformation in how I eat and how I think about food – a transformation for the better. Over time, I have read countless books, magazines, and websites in an effort to understand and learn about how what we put in our bodies impacts our well-being, how our traditional food choices developed, and where the food we eat comes from. Like many people, I used to eat a standard American diet and felt really lousy most of the time. I recall being constantly hungry, often irritable, and either hyperactive or exhausted. I also really knew nothing about the process by which my food reached my plate. Over the years, though, I made gradual changes in my eating habits, I have learned a lot, and I can say that I am a healthier and happier person because of it. For the past decade, I have been maintaining a completely vegan diet – that is, 100% plant-based. My husband is also vegan, and we are raising our little boy vegan as well. I have many reasons for believing that veganism is the best lifestyle choice you can make for yourself and your family, and it seems that as time goes on, more and more people agree!

Most of us are accustomed to eating based on the way we were brought up or based on what is most convenient. It's something that few of us really think much about. But, don't you think we should think about it? We should all care about our well-being and about how what we are putting into our bodies affects us. You and your body are partners in life, and you need to take care of it so it will take care of you.

The amount of information out there on this subject can be extremely overwhelming. Every time I want to suggest a good book on going vegan to a family member or friend, I realize that all the great books I love are simply too long and too detailed for most people who haven't already made a commitment to changing their habits. Let's face it. Just because you love somebody doesn't mean you will read a 500 page book based on their suggestion. However, you might be willing to read a 60 page book. That is why I've written this short handbook on the basics of going vegan.

I think that I have gotten a good handle on the common themes among the opinions of the many experts I admire, and I have condensed all my studying down to some simple concepts that enable me to make the right food choices every day. I have also tried so many different vegan "convenience foods" and done so much cooking that I've picked up some valuable lessons. So, now that I am confident that I eat and feed my family in a healthy, delicious, and practical way, I want to share my knowledge with others. If you are interested in trying out veganism but don't know where to start, this book is for you. Or maybe you already tried going vegan but couldn't stick to it or weren't sure if it was right for you. This book can help you succeed.

I want you to consider this book a launching pad. I can't guarantee that my words will change your life. Only you have the power to do that. I can say that my husband and I do feel many positive effects from living as vegans. I hope that after trying some of my suggestions you will start enjoying a new vegan lifestyle, or that I will at least inspire you to seek out more answers.

So, take the plunge, and read this book with an open mind. When it comes to your health and well-being, ignorance is not bliss. Are you ready for a change?

WHAT IS A HEALTHY VEGAN DIET?

It is extremely easy to describe a healthy vegan diet. It comes down to one sentence that everyone should memorize:

To be a healthy vegan, eat the widest possible variety of minimally processed plant-based foods.

It is as simple as that, but let me elaborate to make it perfectly clear. All whole grains, fruits, vegetables, beans, seeds, nuts, herbs, spices, and unadulterated plant oils are great. These are the foods you can and should eat in abundance. In contrast, animal-based foods are to be avoided. A vegan diet is completely plant-based and contains no animal products. That means no meat, no animal milk, and no eggs. Processed and refined foods should not be consumed excessively. In other words, take it easy on the sugar, white flour (in white bread and pasta, for example), and white rice. You should also not rely too heavily on pre-packaged, processed foods. Trust me that this is not as difficult to put into practice as it may sound at first.

People tend to worry about giving up animal products. They wonder, "What will I eat?" Trust me that living on plant-based foods is not about limiting and depriving yourself. On the contrary, you will probably learn about many great foods that you had no idea existed. Learning to eat a healthy vegan diet is going to give you more options – not fewer. You just have to be open to the possibilities, and you might be surprised at everything you've been missing.

The basics
- Eat lots of: whole grains, fruits, vegetables, beans, seeds, nuts, herbs, spices
- Do not eat any: meat, animal milk, eggs
- Limit: sugar, salt, processed food, white flour, white rice, and white pasta

WHY GO VEGAN?

The primary focus of this book is improving your physical health through choosing veganism. However, the benefit to your own health is only one reason to live on whole, plant-based foods. There are really four broad reasons I want to touch upon:

For the...	*Animals*
For the...	*Earth*
For your...	*Body*
For your...	*Mind*

The choice to change your eating habits may be driven by only one or two of these main reasons, but no matter your initial motivation for giving up animal-based foods, eventually, each of these concepts will play a role in sticking to your commitment. It's about more than just staying healthy (though that's a big part of it). It's about a better life all around – for all of us!

For the... Animals

It is beyond the scope of this book to go into a lengthy discussion of the treatment of animals in the modern farming industry, but I do want to share some thoughts on the matter and a few facts.

I truly feel that the vast majority of people are uncomfortable with the thought of animals suffering. Most of us would not intentionally cause an animal pain. I know that when I still ate meat, I occasionally spared a fleeting thought for the animal whose flesh I was consuming, but I would always push such thoughts out of my mind quickly. I really didn't want to think about it too hard, and, though I may be naïve, I think most people are like me in that way. They have always eaten meat, it's the culturally normal and convenient thing to do, and they try not to think about it too hard. It's also significant that the average person is extremely sheltered from the truth of where our food comes from. We see meat cut up into small, clean pieces wrapped in cellophane in the supermarket or made into burgers, and it's easy to forget what it really is and what has to happen for it to reach that form. The animal agriculture industry itself is, of course, partly responsible for the typical American mindset because of the vast resources they pour into marketing their products, concealing their practices, and convincing people through advertising campaigns that the consumption of animal products is the only way to survive.

> *De-beaking refers to the chopping off of 1/2 to 2/3 of a bird's beak with a hot blade. This causes the chicken to live its life with chronic pain and sensitivity. This apparently prevents it from pecking its neighbors to death.*

The truth of the matter is that modern animal agriculture is shockingly cruel. The picture that comes to mind when we think of the word "farm" is very outdated. In the last 40 to 50 years, the whole industry of producing animals for human consumption has changed. Modern farming techniques are geared only towards streamlining production and increasing profit. Animals raised for meat, milk, and eggs are forced to live in so-called "factory farms" under the most squalid conditions, and they endure tremendous pain and misery throughout their shortened lives. At birth, chickens are de-beaked and piglets have their tails docked, ears notched, testicles removed, and teeth clipped all without the use of anesthetic. These procedures are done to minimize the damage the animals are able to do to each other as they go insane from confinement and attack their neighboring companions. They are crammed by the thousands into spaces that are much too small where many slowly die of disease or lack of access to food and water. The dead are often cannibalized by the other desperate animals. They are bred to grow unnaturally large and in addition are fed a diet meant to fatten them quickly. This causes the animals to suffer great discomfort ranging from the inability to move to the failure of their organs. Slaughtering is a violent, inhumane procedure. Due to the speed with which animals are "processed", many wind up being boiled alive or bleeding to death as their limbs are cut off one by one while the animal is still conscious. Volumes have been written containing descriptions of the conditions in modern factory farms, but it all comes down to this: the lives and deaths of the animals America uses for food are full of pain and intense suffering.

> *Pigs are known to be as sensitive and intelligent as the average household dog. However, the violence perpetrated against them is extreme. 'Tail docking' is the cutting off of the tail right at the base. 'Ear notching' is performed with scissors to create an identifying mark. 'Tooth clipping' is the removal of the incisors with pliers. Castration is done by slicing the scrotum open and reaching in and yanking out the testicles by hand. All of these procedures are done completely without anesthetic.*

I'd like to draw special attention to the plight of the common dairy cow. Many people who are vegetarians for ethical reasons still consume dairy products because of the belief that cows are not harmed in the production of milk. In fact, nothing could be further from the truth. Over the years, the dairy industry has determined that the way to get the greatest milk output from each cow is to artificially impregnate her once a year. This creates a cycle in which each dairy cow gives birth, is milked beginning the next day, is impregnated again three months later, and continues to be milked for seven more months. The cow then does not produce milk for the last two months of the nine-month pregnancy. Once she gives birth, the cycle begins again. In this way, milk production per year is kept as high as possible. Cows treated in this way are exhausted and depleted after about four or five years and are then made into cheap ground beef and pet food. There has been an uproar over the practices of slaughterhouses that butcher the so-called "spent" dairy cows. An undercover investigation by the Humane Society of the United States documented a case in California in which dairy cows that were too weak and ill to even stand – much less walk – were horrifically abused to get them on their feet. Tactics employed by employees included: kicking, ramming with a forklift, jabbing in the eyes, applying electrical shocks, and torturing with a water hose. Much of the meat produced in this slaughterhouse went into the federal school lunch program. What people don't seem to realize is that abuse like this is widespread and has been going on for years. You may well wonder what happens to the many calves produced by the dairy industry. Well, the females are often kept to add to the dairy's stock. The males are sold to the veal industry – well-known to be one of the cruelest industries there is. Calves that are born too small or sickly to be profitable are immediately killed and processed into the low-grade veal used in TV dinners and at cheaper restaurants. Cows are sensitive creatures that form very strong bonds between mother and child. Every dairy cow mourns the loss of every calf taken away from her within a day of birth and never allowed a drop of its mother's milk. Farmers report that the cows bellow for days following each separation.

> *Slaughterhouses operate on the assembly line model. A typical beef plant kills 250 cattle per hour. The workers are completely overwhelmed by the speed of the line, and it is therefore impossible to assure that each animal is rendered unconscious before being hung upside down by the rear legs, having his or her throat cut and belly sliced open. Sometimes animals are fully conscious all the way to the point of having their hides ripped off their bodies.*

If you have thought about eating organic, pasture-raised, cage-free, grass-fed, hormone-free, antibiotic-free animal products precisely because you feel concern for animals, you need to know that all these labels mean very little. I encourage you to look into it further, but I have learned that even farms operating under these terms are full of animal mistreatment. And, no matter what it says on the label, that animal did not willingly go to a peaceful slaughter, and that cow whose milk you are consuming did not willingly give up her offspring to the meat industry.

So ask yourself if you want to contribute to this pain and suffering. Are you really comfortable with the fact that for you to have the food you think you need like burgers, chicken sandwiches, deli subs, scrambled eggs, or even the milk you pour on your cereal, animals have to suffer unspeakable cruelty? Does it seem right to you that over 2,000 land animals die for each human lifetime in this country? Do you really think that these animals do not suffer pain and anguish? Would you protest if 10 billion dogs and cats were treated and slaughtered the way farm animals are? If so, what makes the farm animals so different that they shouldn't be entitled to the same protections as dogs and cats? Yes that's right, 10 billion farm animals are killed for food in the U.S. alone – every year. I know it's hard to face the prospect of changing your habits, and it took me a long time to do it, but do you want to be someone who goes through life with blinders on – just going along with the way things are, or do you want to be aware of the impact your choices have? I finally got to the point where I could not ignore the facts any longer, and I think that if most people really knew the facts and were willing to face them, we would start to make what John Robbins calls, "a cultural shift towards a plant-based diet". Just because humans have used and abused animals for our own purposes for thousands of years doesn't mean it is right. Don't forget that society used to accept slavery, racism, sexism as natural too. Some cultures still do! If you've never thought about it before, perhaps you should. Why not be a proud member of the small group starting the evolution towards a "cultural shift" in how we regard animals?

If this brief discussion of modern animal farming has sparked even the smallest twinge of concern in you, I suggest you read more on the subject and become an educated consumer. The meat, dairy, and egg industries depend on their consumers remaining uninformed.

For the... earth

Research has proven that the raising of cattle and the fishing industry are both disastrous to the environment.

The raising of livestock has virtually decimated the American west. Beef cattle are allowed to graze on approximately 70% of the land in the west – roughly 525 million acres – before they are transported to spend the end of their lives in the factory farms described previously. This has led to a decline in the diversity of natural plant and animal life throughout a vast region of the country. One effect is that through loss of habitat and outright slaughter, our country is completely losing its native wild animals. By the government's own admission, 200,000 wild animals including bears, bobcats, foxes, mountain lions, coyotes, and prairie dogs are killed per year by the U.S. Animal Damage Control Bureau (recently renamed as "Wildlife Services" for obvious public relations reasons). This is done only to protect the interests of cattle ranchers who wield extreme political power. Also, the amount of land we use for growing cattle feed and hay eclipses the amount of land we use to feed people. Because crops are not rotated, this land becomes depleted and less productive every year. If this land was used in a sustainable way to grow food for human consumption, the United States could grow enough good food for the whole world.

Another environmental problem is the waste produced by the animal farming industry. In one incident in North Carolina, 25 million gallons of putrefying hog waste spilled into a river, polluting 364,000 acres of coastal wetlands, killing approximately 12 million fish outright and destroying the breeding areas of half of all middle east coast fish species. For some perspective, the Exxon-Valdez oil spill was 12 million gallons – less than half the amount. But, which disaster got more media coverage?

Fishing also does extreme harm to the environment. We are plundering the oceans of species that are vital to the earth's food chain, and the effects of this are devastating to the planet. It is not only the species that are eaten by humans that are in danger. In order for commercial fishing operations to catch the fish they want, they wind up hauling in and throwing back into the water a great deal of untargeted marine life known in the industry as "bycatch". These dead and dying animals "mistakenly" snared by the fishing nets greatly outnumber the fish actually brought to market. Animals commonly killed in this way include: dolphins, whales, porpoises, sea turtles, birds of various kinds, and many, many fish species.

There is another example of fishing-related violence that I find particularly disturbing. In order to attempt to restore cod populations (decimated by years of over-fishing) off the coast of eastern Canada, fishermen are permitted by the Canadian government to kill approximately 300,000 seals per year. They kill baby and adult harp seals and hood seals. In fact, it has been shown that cod are not even a major source of food for these seals. They are simply being scapegoated in order to appease and employ the out-of-work fishermen, giving them income from the sale of the seal pelts. Not only is this damaging to the seal populations, but, in an ironic twist, there is evidence that these mass seal killings lead to an overgrowth of a certain bacteria in the ocean waters that renders them unable to support marine life of any kind. See www.protectseals.org for more information.

Known as "aquaculture", fish farming is not any less damaging to the environment. Firstly, in order to feed carnivorous species of farmed fish, small wild-caught fish are used thereby disrupting the balance of the food chain. Secondly, coastal fish farms have a very high incidence of disease due to the crowded conditions, and these diseases easily spread to the open sea through the water itself or through the many fish that escape the farms.

I hope the information presented here makes it clear that the consumption of animal-based foods is inconsistent with being environmentally conscious.

For your... body
Most people, if pressed, would say that they'd prefer to live a long and healthy life over the alternative. However, eating a diet high in animal protein has been shown to be directly related to some of the modern world's deadliest conditions including cancer, obesity, diabetes, and heart disease.

Animal milk and products made from it (like cheese and ice cream) are high in saturated fats. These are the fats that build up in our bodies and cause blocking of the arteries and heart disease. Dairy cows are given hormones to keep them lactating at full capacity and antibiotics to keep them alive and free of the infections they are prone to acquire from being hooked up to machinery all day and from living in close, unsanitary conditions. When we consume dairy products, these hormones and antibiotics enter our own bodies where they affect our reproductive and immune systems. Even the dairy industry's claims about milk being the best calcium source are simply untrue. The reason cow's milk naturally contains calcium is because traditionally, cows got calcium from eating grass. Modern dairy cows, however, now have calcium added artificially to their feed since they spend their lives in feedlots with no access to grass. You would do better to get your calcium from just eating leafy green vegetables and/or consuming fortified foods (like enriched, organic soymilk). There is no reason for getting your calcium second-hand out of a cow. There are even studies that show that eating animal-based foods causes the human body to actually lose calcium leading to bone weakness. In all, cow's milk consumption has been linked to: cancer, diabetes, obesity, heart disease, and osteoporosis.

Animal meat is also an unhealthy substance for humans. We are often told that we must eat meat to get enough protein in our diet. Protein is indeed an essential substance for our bodies. Science has not been able to pinpoint exactly why, but the fact is that the human body needs protein in order to survive. Studies have shown, though, that typical Americans regularly consume up to double the daily recommended protein intake because of all the animal products we consume. Too much protein in the diet can lead to serious health problems. As mentioned above, excess protein can cause your body to lose calcium. This can lead to bone loss and even osteoporosis. Also, when you consume more protein than your body needs, a complex reaction begins. The excess protein causes ammonia to be released by your cells. This ammonia turns to urea that has to be processed by the liver and kidneys – organs essential to cleaning the blood of impurities. This is actually a lot of extra work for those organs, causing dehydration as a short term effect and the possibility of kidney and liver weaknesses in the long term. The truth is that all foods contain protein. Beans, nuts, and whole grains are especially protein-rich. We can get our full requirement of healthy protein by eating these foods and will also avoid the problems associated with protein over-consumption.

Beef, pork, and poultry are the main sources of meat in the U.S. Most of these meats contain hormones, antibiotics, and pesticide residues from the food the animals are given. These substances, harmful as they may be, can be avoided by choosing organic meats. However, organic meat – like regular meat – contains unhealthy levels of saturated fat and cholesterol no matter how lean the cut. It is well documented that meat consumption has been and continues to be heavily implicated in many incidences of heart disease and blood vessel disorders as well as colon cancer. The other problem with meat is what I mentioned before about the way it is processed and the way the animals are kept in close confinement in very unsanitary conditions. There is just nothing appetizing about the meat industry. Even the feed given to farm animals partially consists of byproducts from the processing of their own kind. This can lead to serious health implications such as mad cow (a disease affecting the brain in a way similar to Alzheimer's) and foot and mouth disease (a severe, incurable, highly contagious, viral infection that cannot, however, be passed to humans). Shoddy, assembly-line butchering leaves a lot of room for mistakes, including the introduction of dangerous bacteria like E. coli into the meat. This leads to huge numbers of food poisoning cases in this country. It is estimated that there are anywhere from 20 to 80 million cases of severe, meat-related food-borne illnesses in the U.S. per year. In another frightening development, it is now a common practice to inject meat with carbon monoxide gas in order to keep it looking bright red and fresh long after it would have otherwise turned gray. The carbon monoxide itself is considered safe by the FDA, but it is very problematic that meat treated with it appears fresh when it may not be. How can you avoid spoiled meat if you can't see that it is spoiled? The practice has been banned in the European Union, but is common in the U.S. Also, it is common knowledge that carbon monoxide is a carcinogen. I would rather not consume it even at so-called safe levels.

Even fish – the so-called healthy alternative to meat – is not a good food source. Unfortunately, the polluted state of our oceans causes high concentrations of chemicals such as mercury and other dangerous substances to accumulate in the flesh of fish. Much of the salmon, trout, cod, tilapia, and shrimp sold in stores and served in restaurants today is actually farm-raised. Farmed fish live either in tanks or in areas of ocean along a shoreline that are contained with net-like barriers. Many of these farmed fish are genetically modified for various traits (like color and size), and their conditions can be quite unsanitary since there is typically not enough water to support the number of fish raised in a given area. In addition to the effects of poor sanitation, genetic modification, and chemical pollution, there is the fact that like all meat, fish is high in saturated fat and cholesterol. It is widely said that fish is the best source of Omega 3 fatty acids essential for skin health, a strong immune system, and more, but actually, you can get plenty of Omega 3's from flax seeds, flax oil, and leafy green vegetables such as spinach, kale, and chard with none of the ill effects common from eating fish.

Not surprisingly, eggs also have a high saturated fat and cholesterol content and have the strong tendency to contain harmful bacteria such as salmonella. As with dairy cows, egg laying hens are pumped full of antibiotics and hormones that eventually wind up in the eggs we eat.

In contrast to all the information above, plant foods have no adverse effect on health or unappealing sources of origin. On the contrary, the more you eat fruits, vegetables, nuts, seeds, and grains you eat, the more health benefits your body receives from your food in the form of vitamins, minerals, fiber, anti-oxidants, and essential fats. Pound for pound, plant foods are much richer in these substances than animal-based foods. So, not only are animal products bad for you in a direct way, but also every time you eat them, you are displacing the more nutritious plant foods out of your diet. Did you know, for example, that animal foods are completely devoid of fiber? When you fill up on them, you prevent yourself from consuming the plant foods that aid your digestive system and keep it running smoothly. The healthier your digestive system is, the lower your risk of getting colon and stomach cancer. Did you also know that meat takes up to two weeks to pass through your system whereas whole, plant-based foods take 24 hours or less? Think about it. Do you really want your steak dinner to be sitting inside you for that long? So, overall, the more animal products you consume, the fewer nutrients you get and the higher your chances of developing a life-threatening illness.

For your... mind

This last of the broad reasons for living a lifestyle free of animal based foods is a bit more abstract and may not apply to everyone. However, because this aspect has been very important to me, I want to explain how my mental and emotional well-being has been greatly affected by my dietary choices.

Each time I have improved my lifestyle to omit the consumption or use of an animal-based product, I have felt a palpable brightening of my spirit. I've wondered about the cause of this, and I can only assume that I must have felt a certain subconscious guilt all along. And, yes, any guilt was subconscious. I never consciously thought that there was anything wrong with eating animals and their milk and eggs.

As my habits have changed, though, I have definitely felt the gradual lifting of a weight off me.

When I stopped eating animals, I noticed that I felt a bit more at peace with nature and that when I saw a picture or image of a cow, chicken, turkey, or pig, I could smile and feel a kinship with the animal that I lacked before. As children we are raised to find these animals cute and we learn to mimic their oinking, mooing, clucking, and gobbling. At some point, though, in order to become comfortable with the concept of eating them, we cease to think of these animals as having any special merit, and in my opinion, that is a great loss. When we stop eating them, we can recover the sense of joy and wonder we had as children upon contemplating them. Their lives become no less meaningful than a dog's or a cat's or a horse's or even a human's, and it feels wonderful to be able to appreciate them again as the lovely, comical, peaceful, and fascinating creatures they are. Upon becoming a vegetarian, Franz Kafka wrote, "Now I can at last look at you in peace. I don't eat you anymore." I know exactly what he meant. Of course there is also pain associated with waking up to the animals' suffering and seeing others continue to consume them, but this is balanced by the pride and peace of mind I feel from knowing that they no longer suffer and die for me. If you are the kind of person who instinctively says, "I love animals," you will get a powerful sense of peace when you begin to live in harmony with your true feelings.

One of the greatest things about raising my son vegan is that I can teach him about the animals and the noises they make without feeling like I am at the same time feeding him those animals without his knowledge. I'll never forget the time I gave my 7 year old niece a veggie burger. She asked, "If this burger is made from veggies, what are other burgers made from?" I told her as gently as possible that they were made from cows' bodies. She absolutely did not believe me! She had to confirm it with her parents. I think that, given the option, a child would not knowingly consume dead animals if they had other tasty food to choose from.

If you consider yourself a non-violent and peaceful person, you should know that choosing to not eat animals is the single most effective thing you can do to reduce violence in the world. There is a real correlation between violence to animals and violence to people, and there is an undeniable connection between the violence perpetrated in the slaughterhouse and the meat on your plate. Violence is pervasive in our society, and whether it is against animals, people, or property, it all comes from the same mindset. If you say you don't believe in violence, and you feel ineffectual and like there is nothing you can do to change the world, I want you to know that this is something that you can do. It does make a difference, and it will make you feel better... guaranteed.

My sense of peace and harmony with the earth and all her creatures has intensified as I have learned to omit all animal products from my life. Not only do I not eat animal products anymore, but I have also stopped purchasing clothing made from animal products (such as leather, wool, and goose down), and I only buy personal care products that were not tested on animals and that contain no animal byproducts. (For example, most bar soap contains animal fat.) It is difficult to explain, but the knowledge that I no longer mindlessly support businesses that profit from animal suffering has really made a positive impact on me. I know that many other people have experienced this same phenomenon when they make the shift to a lifestyle free of animal-based products.

THE NEXT STEP

After reading the information presented so far, you are now faced with a choice. This is where you have to be really honest with yourself and make a decision. Are you willing to begin the process of making changes in your life? Will you continue with the habits you've had and the food choices you've made until now, or are you ready to question, to know what you are eating and drinking, to reap the benefits of a healthy diet, to live a better life? That's really what it comes down to. I have spoken to numerous people about the issues set forth above. Often, people will say that they understand and believe all of it. They may even go so far as to agree that the "right" thing to do would be to go vegan. However, many people are just not ready or willing to consider change, and that is the end of it. Maybe you don't really care about your health, you don't believe animals have the capacity to feel pain, you don't think the environment is your responsibility, you don't believe me or my sources, or maybe you just like meat too much and are set in your ways. Those are all, sadly, unfortunate points of view, but if that's you, then there isn't much more I can say. I wish everyone was willing to change, but I know that only a few people are.

The rest of this book is for those of you who have been inspired to try to change or are curious about a new way of life. By just being willing to try, you are going to take a giant step towards a happier, healthier life. You don't have to change everything all at once. Any change you make in the direction of living on a wholesome plant-based diet will improve your life. As you begin to feel the effects of better choices, it will get easier and easier to make even more good choices. You should look at it as a process and not a scary event that has to happen instantly. I'm going to try to make it as easy as possible for you to get started. I want you to learn from my experiences, and I want you to have fun learning new habits. All you have to do is be willing to keep reading, be ready to try something new, and I will help you take it from there.

YOUR NEW MENU

I'm sure some of you eat the same way I used to: coffee and a donut or muffin for breakfast (maybe a bacon, egg, and cheese sandwich), pizza, a burger, or a deli sandwich for lunch, sugary and/or salty highly-processed snacks throughout the day, and a dinner consisting of meat, something starchy like white rice or pasta, and a token vegetable or two slathered in butter. Oh, and don't forget the soda, coffee, and alcoholic beverages with very little if any straight water. The bad news is that there is practically nothing redeeming about this diet at all. This typical day's intake is high in sugar and sodium, high in calories, high in saturated fat and cholesterol, overly high in protein, low in vitamins and minerals, and low in fiber.

Now, I want to be honest with you and let you know that I do understand that there is some adjustment involved here. However, I also know that with a small amount of effort up front, you can be setting yourself up for years and years of feeling much better than you might have otherwise. Trust me when I say that all the changes I recommend are really not hard to keep up with once you get used to them. I guarantee that your tastes will adjust, your habits will adjust, and this can all be done painlessly. Positive results you can expect to experience include: increased lifespan, healthy weight, decreased stress, increased energy, and a general sense of well-being and peace of mind. Oh, and please get out of your head the notion that living a plant-based lifestyle is equal to deprivation. By following my suggestions, you get to experience countless foods that you may not have otherwise even considered. Not only that, but you can eat as much of these foods as you want. This is the opposite of deprivation – it's called abundance. In fact, the best way to approach this is simply to start trying the new, healthy, and delicious foods I recommend throughout this chapter. As you fill up on these new foods, they begin to displace the unhealthy and animal-based foods you currently eat. Eventually you no longer crave the foods you used to. Like I said before, treat this as a process. This way you will never feel that you are giving things up, but rather that you are expanding your choices.

Where to shop

I have found that the very best place to shop is Whole Foods Market. They have the best selection of all-natural, vegan foods, their produce is excellent, and their store-brand products and bulk, self-service area are economical and offer a lot of great vegan products. Many people think Whole Foods is an expensive place to shop, but that is more because the quality of the food there is higher. You do get what you pay for. If you are not able to shop at Whole Foods, though, no fear. Most supermarkets these days are carrying lots of natural foods and meat substitutes. Find out whether there is a health food store in your area that you can use to pick up the things you can't find at the local supermarket. And, of course, there is always the internet!

Things to keep in mind

- Don't focus on "giving up" foods.
- Just start trying new, healthy, delicious foods.
- This leaves less room for your usual fare.
- Eventually, you will see that the new foods are delicious and make you feel better, and you will cease to crave the old foods.

Your new food groups

Grains

Unfortunately, most of us are in the nasty habit of eating only refined grains that have been stripped of most of their vitamins, minerals, and fiber. We eat white bread, white rice, white pasta, and baked goods made with white flour. The reason these foods are white is because they have been highly processed. The most nutrient-rich portions of the wheat and rice grains have been removed. Until the late 1800's everyone ate whole grains all the time. Then, a process was developed to remove portions of the grain. The resulting product was considered superior because of its smooth texture and white color. At the time, it also seemed healthier because mold and fungus became less likely to contaminate the stored grain. However, all these white, processed foods are full of empty calories and carbohydrates, and by eating them you are missing out on a great opportunity to fortify your diet with the many nutrients in whole grain foods. By simply changing most of the bread, cereal, pasta, and rice you eat to whole grain versions of these foods that use full, unprocessed grains, you can lower your caloric intake, feel more satisfied with less food (because these foods tend to be heartier and more filling than their processed counterparts), and receive huge health benefits -- from lowering your cholesterol levels to improving your digestive function. I will admit to using some white flour when I bake desserts. I think that using it in this way is fine as long as you are using whole grains in the majority of foods you eat throughout the day. The point is to increase your whole grain to refined grain ratio as much as you can. Getting a variety of nutritious whole grains in your diet is very easy but may require you to expand your horizons a bit initially.

Bread
In terms of bread, you are going to want to go for whole wheat or whole grain whenever possible. Please take a look at the label of the bread you buy. One unfortunate fact is that most whole wheat bread contains high fructose corn syrup which is a completely unnecessary, highly refined and processed sweetener. Also, you will often find that only some of the flour used is whole grain, and there will still be white flour included. It is worth trying several brands to figure out which you like best. The store-brand bread (especially whole wheat and 12

grain, organic or not) at Whole Foods is excellent. My absolute favorite is Vermont Bread Company. Their "Soft Whole Wheat" and "Soft Whole Grain" sandwich breads are absolutely wonderful and free of questionable additives. Rudi's Organic brand is also great. These breads can be found in many supermarkets, but you may have to go to your local health food store if your supermarket doesn't carry them.

Cereals

With breakfast cereals, you should also read labels carefully. Even if a cereal claims to be whole grain on the front of the box, it could be full of additives and skimpy on the grains. Be especially careful of sugar content. Sugar can be listed as many things in an ingredient list. One of the most common ways it is listed is as high fructose corn syrup. Avoid this ingredient at all costs. Also, many cereals contain milk products! I particularly love all the Cascadian Farm cereals. Kashi cereals are quite good, though the ones I particularly like are "Strawberry Fields", "Oat Flakes and Blueberry Clusters", and "Cinnamon Harvest". I am also a big fan of Nature's Path "Maple Pecan Crunch". Granolas can also be very good sources of grain. Again, read your labels. The high nut content in some granolas can make it seem like the fat content is very high, but these are fats that are good for the body. Hot cereals are one of the best sources of whole grains. Just about any grain can be cooked up into a delicious and satisfying breakfast cereal. My personal favorites for the morning are oats, quinoa, or barley. The oats are best cooked by the serving (I buy organic quick oats in bulk at Whole Foods), but with any whole grain you can make batches you keep in the fridge for a quick, easily prepared breakfast. I like cooking my grains with water as described on the package and putting them into a container in the fridge. Then, when it's time for breakfast, place a cup of cooked grain in a bowl, add some non-dairy milk, maple syrup, cinnamon, and fruit (like blueberries or a chopped banana).

You can simmer this until warmed through or even microwave it if you are in a hurry. Of course there are many hot cereals available on the market to simplify matters, but again be careful of added sugar, artificial flavorings, and other additives. If you do go for a commercial hot cereal, you can pick anything made by Bob's Red Mill or Arrowhead Mills. Both of those companies make a wide variety of whole grain hot cereals that are delicious and healthy.

Rice and other grains

Instead of eating white rice as a side dish, consider brown rice (I prefer short grain) or one of the many other whole grains that are cooked in the same way as rice: pearled barley, bulgur wheat, millet, quinoa, or a wild rice blend. All of these grains are delicious and nutty and so much more nutritious than white rice. They also leave you much more satisfied with less quantity. My special favorite is quinoa. It is an ancient South American grain and is chock full of nutrients. You cook it just like rice with a 1 cup grain to 2 cups water ratio. One special thing to note about quinoa is that you should always rinse it thoroughly in a sieve first before cooking. Otherwise, the final product can be somewhat bitter. As long as you give the grain a quick rinse first, though, it has a wonderful flavor and fluffy texture. Also, polenta or whole wheat couscous are wonderful grain side-dishes.

Pasta

These days it is even easy to find whole grain pasta. This pasta is chewier than regular pasta in the same way that brown rice is chewier than white rice. It isn't a sin to occasionally eat some regular white pasta, but if you tend to eat it very frequently, it is really worth substituting whole wheat pasta at least some of the time. Alternatives to wheat pasta are now easy to find too including, quinoa, spelt, and kamut pastas.

Please note that almost all dry pasta is vegan, and almost all fresh pasta has egg. So, stick with dried.

Vegetables

Everything I've read is in agreement that you can't go wrong by eating vegetables. The FDA recommends 2½ cups per day, but I would take that as a minimum. For the purposes of this book, by the way, I'm not including beans in the vegetable category but rather in the protein category.

Some vegetables are more beneficial to our bodies than others in terms of their concentration of nutrients. Some of the veggies considered to be among the most nutritious are: dark leafy greens (like spinach or kale), onions, garlic, ginger, carrots, bell peppers, shiitake mushrooms, tomatoes, sweet potatoes, beets, broccoli, and seaweed. I encourage you to eat some dark green vegetable plus at least one other every day. You will be ensuring that your body gets the widest variety of vitamins and minerals from whole food sources. It is best to consume vegetables fresh and minimally cooked. You really want to stay away from canned vegetables because of their typically high sodium content and the fact that many of their nutrients have leeched out. Even in frozen vegetables some nutrients are lost, though frozen is definitely better than canned and can really help when you are trying to make dinner quickly. Go for organic frozen veggies whenever possible.

Speaking of organic vegetables, the problem with non-organic produce is that it contains residue from the pesticides and chemical fertilizers used in its farming. There is concern that these substances may cause cancer. Non-organic produce can also be genetically modified, and little is known about the effects of genetic manipulation on nutrition. I have learned, though, that there are certain crops that traditionally contain the highest concentration of chemicals and are most often genetically manipulated, so if you go organic even for just those specific foods, you can almost completely eliminate your consumption of harmful substances. So, if you are limited in how often you can go organic (either by budget or by availability), at least do purchase organic varieties of these particular veggies: bell peppers, spinach, potatoes, celery, corn, and lettuces.

Fruits

As with vegetables, you are free to really go to town with fresh fruit. The FDA recommends 2 cups a day, and again, I say to use that as a starting point. One way I frequently get my whole daily fruit requirement in one go is to make a smoothie containing a banana and one cup of frozen berries. One of those each day, and you're all set! But, you definitely want to eat a wide variety of fruits. Some fruits that have particularly great health benefits are: blueberries, oranges, bananas, and apples. I recommend getting through that whole list each week and trying other fruits whenever you can. Go for fresh as often as possible, but frozen or dried fruit is great too.

By the way, fruit juices (even those that are 100% pure and natural) are not a good substitute for eating whole fruits. They are missing the beneficial fiber in the fruit and have a higher concentration of naturally-occurring sugars. However, dried fruits with no sugar added definitely count towards your fruit consumption.

The fruits for which you should really stick to organic are: peaches, apples, nectarines, strawberries, cherries, pears, and grapes or raisins. Again, there is great organic frozen fruit for those times when eating fresh fruit isn't practical. Frozen berries are especially convenient for adding to hot cereals, non-dairy yogurt, pancakes, and smoothies.

Fats

You might think it is necessary to avoid all fat, but this isn't true. The fats that are particularly unhealthy are basically the saturated fats and trans-fats. Saturated fats are solid at room temperature and include animal fats as well as coconut oil and palm oil. Trans fats are usually unsaturated fats that have had hydrogen added to them artificially, thereby making them more saturated. They are listed on ingredient labels as hydrogenated or partially hydrogenated oils. Monounsaturated fats and Omega-3 fatty acids are the most beneficial and necessary fats. By preparing your meals with healthy oils and eating nuts and seeds at snack time, you will help your body fight and treat disease, you will better absorb nutrients from fruits and vegetables, and you will consume disease-fighting antioxidants.

The best oil-based sources of monounsaturated fats and Omega-3 fatty acids are: extra-virgin olive, canola, peanut, and flaxseed. Flaxseed oil should only be used raw – not in cooking – and needs to be refrigerated. It is wonderful drizzled over veggies instead of butter or used to make salad dressing. Canola oil works in any dish calling for oil. Extra virgin olive oil is best in dishes that will be enhanced but not overpowered by its robust flavor. Peanut oil tends to be best in Asian dishes. All of these oils should be used only in moderation, however, as they do not qualify as "whole foods". Too much oil especially if combined with too little exercise can lead to weight gain.

Add nuts, nut butters and seeds to your diet as well for a whole food source of healthy fats. The best nuts are: macadamias, hazelnuts, pecans, almonds, walnuts, and cashews. The best seeds are flax seeds, sesame seeds, and pumpkin seeds. These nuts and seeds contain the best ratios of healthy fats and the most vitamins and minerals. Eat nuts raw rather than roasted whenever possible for the maximum nutritional value, and try to stick with unsalted. Buy ground flax seeds (or grind them yourself), sprinkle them on cereal, and put a spoonful in your smoothies. Sesame seeds can be sprinkled over lots of different foods, and pumpkin seeds can be eaten along with the nuts as a snack. Peanut butter is a good fat too, but be careful to buy an organic one. Peanuts are among the most highly pesticide-contaminated crops. Also, the very best peanut butter has only one ingredient: peanuts. Added salt and sugar is absolutely unnecessary and unhealthy. I highly recommend Arrowhead Mills or the Whole Foods store brand. Almond butter and cashew butter are also delicious and are good alternatives to peanut butter for something different.

Proteins

As I discussed above in the "For your health" section, most people consume much more protein than is necessary. Animal-based products are simply higher in protein than our bodies need, and this leads to all kinds of issues. It is also a myth that vegetarians suffer from protein deficiency. I encourage you to remove meat and eggs completely from your diet for all the reasons that have been mentioned and for many more reasons that you can learn about from other sources. You may want to do this gradually. One way of doing it is eliminating meat from one additional day of the week each month for 7 months. Skip meat on Mondays for the first month, then Mondays and Wednesdays for the second month, etc. Another way is to eliminate one animal per month. Stop consuming pork products first, one month later eliminate beef, then poultry, then seafood. If you feel willing and able to speed up this process, however, go for it! You can stop eating meat overnight with no bad effects as long as you replace it with the right foods.

Okay, so what should you eat to get the appropriate amount of protein for your body? Beans, nuts, seeds, and whole grains are the very best sources of protein. When we eat a variety of these foods, we get all of the high quality protein we need without the health disadvantages of meat. These foods are also very filling and help satisfy our appetites in a healthy way.

All beans are an excellent source of protein, but soy beans are especially good. Soy products like tofu and tempeh are a great way to get your protein in an all-natural whole-food source. These two foods made from soybeans are minimally processed and have been staples for centuries in Asia. They can be used crumbled up, in bite-sized pieces, or in slices to make a variety of dishes. Search the internet for tofu and tempeh recipes and don't be afraid to experiment. People seem to have a fear of tofu. Just be brave, and don't give up until you have figured out how to cook it. There are some companies that help you out by selling pre-baked or pre-seasoned tofu. These are great and convenient, but also much more expensive than buying it plain. It's a good way to start, though. Of course, when buying a pre-seasoned tofu, make sure the ingredients are wholesome and that there isn't too much sodium (see the "Things to Avoid" chapter).

Tofu tips

- When you need sliced or cubed tofu, buy "extra firm" and make sure to press the water out of it. I highly recommend a tofu press such as the TofuXpress or "Tofu Presser". Cut into slices or cubes, toss with seasonings appropriate for the dish, and then broil in a toaster until somewhat browned. This makes the tofu really tasty and chewy and able to stand up to being tossed into a pan with veggies for example.
- Purchase in the refrigerated section (white tubs with plastic on top)

- Whole Foods brand, Nasoya, WestSoy, Wildwood are all good
- Must be organic or at least non-GMO

Tempeh is a fermented soy product and may have more health benefits than tofu. It does require quite a lot of seasoning, so I recommend starting out with pre-flavored varieties.

Tempeh tips
- Find in refrigerated section with tofu and seitan wrapped in vacuum sealed plastic
- Try flavored varieties first

Wonderful beans include: black beans, chick peas, pinto beans, cannellini beans, and lentils. There are countless dishes you can prepare with these beans spanning an array of ethnic cuisines. Again, just search the internet! The least expensive option with beans is to buy them dry and prepare them from scratch. However, I do tend to go for the convenience of canned beans. Just make sure that whenever you use canned beans you drain them and rinse them thoroughly. They will taste better, and you will remove most of the salt that way. Whole Foods brand has organic, no-salt canned beans that are very good.

Seitan is another absolutely fantastic and healthy protein choice. It is made from the most protein-rich part of the wheat berry. You can buy it in health food stores and in some supermarkets. Chopped up, it is excellent in stir fries and in any recipe calling for strips or chunks of meat. It has a much denser and "meatier" texture than tofu.

Seitan tips
- Made from wheat gluten and extremely high in protein
- Neutral tasting with a very chewy, meaty texture

- Cut into chunks or strips for dishes like stir fries or grind up in food processor to put in chili, pasta sauces, tacos etc.
- Buy WestSoy brand in refrigerated section
- OR make your own (best tried after using the store bought stuff for some time and if you are feeling adventurous!)

Whole grains contain a surprising amount of protein as do nuts and seeds. Quinoa is the most protein-rich grain. See the grains and fats sections for more.

As with other plant foods, there are certain things I've mentioned in this section that you really should go with organic options for when possible. Soy beans, any soy product, and peanuts are the ones that are most likely to contain harmful substances or to be genetically modified if you don't go organic. In fact, you may have heard claims that soy is bad for you because of genetic modification. It's true that most soybean crops are genetically modified, but these tend to be the crops destined for farm animal feed -- not human consumption. Even so, go for organic, and you don't have to worry about it.

Now a word about eggs. They may be tasty, but you know by now that they should be avoided. Eggs are much easier to live without than most people realize. Most of the things we think we need eggs to make can be easily made without eggs with no noticeable difference at all. To substitute for eggs in practically any baked good, for example, pour three parts very hot water over 1 part ground flax seeds (Bob's Red Mill is a great brand). Let sit for 3 to 5 minutes and then whisk vigorously. Use a quarter cup of this in place of each egg required. I have gotten amazing results using this method in cakes, cookies, pancakes, etc. There are also plant-based commercial egg replacers that work quite well. Two good brands are Ener-G and Bob's Red Mill. If you like eggs for breakfast, you can try scrambled tofu as an alternative. There are many recipes for it online, and you are sure to find one that will suit you.

Sometimes you may find yourself craving meat. Here's a fact for you: when we think we are craving meat, it is not really the meat we crave, but the fat, salt, flavorings, and textures associated with the meat dishes we are used to. Do you salivate when you see a cow or pig or rabbit? Do you dream of tearing right into it with your teeth? A lion might, but I guarantee that you definitely don't. Humans have no natural requirement for meat. For some of you, though, it will be hard to imagine life without meat at the center of your plate. Tradition and habit are powerful forces, and I'm not going to deny it. If that is your situation, it is perfectly acceptable to occasionally center a meal on imitation meat. The longer you eat healthfully, the more these cravings will fade away, but in the meantime, these products serve a great purpose. As with all processed food, though, read labels carefully for additives and sodium content, and don't center your entire diet on them. Eating them once or twice a week is fine. My recommendations in the chart below are for the imitation meats that I have found to be tastiest without too many unhealthy additives. They are completely plant-based.

Here's a hint: do an internet search for any product you might want to try. Getting an idea of what the package looks like will make it easier to find at the store. All these products will be found in the refrigerated section unless otherwise noted. Some stores put this stuff with the vegetables, and some put it with the dairy. Additionally, some stores have a special natural foods section where you can find these products. Be sure to look thoroughly before deciding your store doesn't carry something. Then, if they really don't, ask them to! All of these products are available at Whole Foods Market as of the writing of this book.

Meat Product	Vegetarian Substitute
Raw Ground Beef	Lightlife Gimme Lean Ground Beef Style
Browned Ground Beef	Lightlife Smart Ground WestSoy Ground seitan Tofurky ground beef style
Beef Strips or Chunks	Lightlife Steak Style Strips Gardein Homestyle Beefless Tips (frozen) WestSoy Seitan
Beef Burgers	Amy's All American Burger (frozen) Boca Original Vegan (frozen) Make from scratch with Gimme Lean
Meatballs	Nate's (frozen) Whole Foods (frozen) Make meatballs with Lightlife Gimme Lean
Chicken Patties or Cutlets	Gardein Chick'n Scalloppini (frozen) Boca Original Chik'n Patties (frozen)
Chicken Strips or Chunks	Lightlife Chick'n Strips Beyond Meat Chicken Free Strips Gardein Chick'n Scalloppini (frozen)
Hot Dogs	Lightlife Tofu Pups
Breakfast Sausage	Field Roast Apple Sage or Apple Maple
Italian Sausage	Lightlife Gimme Lean Sausage Style (crumbled) Tofurkey Artisan line Field Roast Grain Meat Sausages - Italian
Other sausage	Field Roast Smoked Apple Sage Sausage Field Roast Mexican Tofurkey Artisan Spinach Pesto
Bacon	Lightlife Smart Bacon Lightlife Fakin' Bacon tempeh

Deli Meats	Field Roast Deli Slices Tofurkey Deli Slices
Meatloaf	Field Roast Classic Meatloaf Make from Scratch with Gimme Lean
Roasted Turkey	Field Roast Celebration Roast Tofurkey Roast (frozen)

Dairy Substitution

Dairy is a food group that you should eliminate completely from your diet. Most of us grew up hearing that it was good to drink milk and consume dairy products, and as we grew up we never challenged the norm. As I mentioned above, however, even milk's claim to calcium is misleading. There is no good reason to consume milk and plenty of good reasons not to. Here's an interesting fact: 75% of the world's human population is lactose intolerant. Our bodies are simply not meant to digest any species' milk beyond infancy much less cow's milk.

So, just skip the dairy altogether and go for the many delicious plant-based varieties of common dairy products. I find non-dairy butter, yogurt, ice cream, sour cream, and cream cheese to be delicious. For milk, we are lucky to have tons of choices. There is soy milk, almond milk, rice milk, and others. These milks work great in every recipe you can think of that calls for milk. Each type and brand has its own particular taste and thickness, so try a wide variety before you pick a favorite. People sometimes try one soymilk brand, and because they don't fall in love with it, assume they just dislike all plant milks. Do yourself a favor, and don't stop trying them until you find one you like!

Though all these products do contain fat, it is the kind of fat that is good for our bodies. So you can enjoy a texture and flavor similar to creamy, full-fat dairy without the health concerns. An added benefit is that most soy products are also organic, and when you choose those, you know you are getting wholesome, additive-free food. Also, since these products are marketed to the health-conscious, they are often fortified with vitamins and minerals (including calcium and vitamins A, D, B12, and others) to enhance the health benefits. Plus, in most supermarkets, it is getting downright easy to find these foods.

Now I just want to be clear that none of these foods are necessary for a healthy diet. However, since dairy is so ubiquitous in most people's eating habits, I am providing this section to show you some alternatives. You could go without these foods, but if you are hooked on the dairy versions, switching over to these varieties is a great thing you can do to improve your health.

I am going to suggest some specific brands and products that I have chosen as the best and tastiest options. Yes, these are my personal opinions, but believe me, I've tried it all, and I have good reason for picking the products I did. I want to make it as easy as possible for you to try healthy foods without getting overwhelmed by the options. Start incorporating these products into your life. There will be an adjustment period, but if you switch over gradually, and are really committed, you can do it!

So here is my table of common dairy products and the dairy-free substitutes I have found to be the tastiest and healthiest:

Dairy Product	Dairy-Free Substitute
Butter	Earth Balance Buttery Spread
Milk	Whole Foods Brand WestSoy Almond Breeze Dream Blends (highly fortified. Best for kids!) So Delicious
Yogurt	So Delicious Cultured Coconut Milk Almond Dream Yogurt WholeSoy Yogurt
Cream Cheese	Tofutti Better Than Cream Cheese * Get the "Non Hydrogenated Plain"
Sour Cream	Tofutti Better than Sour Cream
Ice Cream	So Delicious (almond, soy, or coconut based)
Cream	Silk Original Creamer So Delicious
Whipped Cream	Soyatoo Soy Whip
Parmesan Cheese	Galaxy Foods Vegan Grated Topping
Mayonnaise	Vegenaise Nayonaise (more like Miracle Whip)

I can't tell you how happy I've been with each one of those products, and I hope you will try them.

No cheese?!

You probably noticed that I did not mention anything about cheeses other than cream cheese and parmesan. I'm not going to lie to you... cheese is a hard habit to break. Almost everyone who goes dairy-free has a hard time giving up cheese, and that's because it is an addictive food, and it happens to be very hard to find a healthy substitute for. Firstly, understand that cheese is something you really should avoid. It is full of unhealthy saturated fat and cholesterol and does nothing for you nutritionally. However, our bodies become physically addicted to the fat and salt content in cheese as well as its texture. If you can completely stop eating it through sheer willpower for a few weeks, I promise you the cravings will go away. Don't let cheese control your life. You are stronger than a piece of cheese! But, I will suggest some things for you to try, if you are really having trouble cutting it completely.

FYI, the soy cheeses that taste most like dairy cheese have large amounts of something called "casein" in them. Casein is a protein extracted from cow's milk, and is heavily implicated in causing cancer. See Dr. T. Colin Campbell's "The China Study" for the proof of this. So, read your labels. If you find a soy cheese with casein or caseinate, then the chances are good that it would satisfy your craving for cheese without the lactose and cholesterol and with less saturated fat. However, do be aware that animal protein forms a large percentage of this product, and it is not a healthy food.

There is such a thing as truly dairy-free cheese. A brand has come out recently called Daiya. I happen to really like it, but I won't lie to you and say you won't be able to tell the difference between it and dairy cheese. One thing you might try is starting to combine Daiya with your dairy cheese, and gradually increase the ratio until you have developed a taste for it.

Daiya Cheese tips
- *Mozzarella Style Shreds*
  Good for melting on Italian dishes
- *Cheddar Style Shreds*
  I like this mixed 50/50 with the mozzarella on Mexican foods.

- *Jack Style Wedge*
  To me, this is the only acceptable vegan cheese to eat on crackers or cold sandwiches. I think it tastes great and has a firm but creamy texture.
- I would steer clear of their other products unless you try and like the above and then feel adventurous. I really only eat these three. I haven't been too impressed with the slices or the other flavors.

There are also some companies that have come out with some artisanal, nut-based cheeses for slicing and spreading. One of these is Kite Hill. These are delicious (albeit expensive) and can be a wonderful addition to your vegan diet if you are inclined to try them. I like that they don't try to emulate cheese exactly but aim to be delicious in their own right!

Drinks

Most people do not consume nearly enough water. The common recommendation is 64 ounces a day which is a half-gallon. This is actually the proper amount for a 128 pound person. The simplest formula is to divide your weight in pounds by two. This gives the ounces of water you need per day. One thing to realize that makes all of this easier is that you don't have to get all 64 (more or less) ounces by drinking straight water. Eating raw fruits and vegetables contributes somewhat towards your fluid intake as do other beverages (such as non-dairy milk and juice) as long as they don't have caffeine or alcohol. As for which kind of water to drink, I've learned that the best choice is tap water that has been run through a filter. I use a water filter that attaches right to the tap. I fill a pitcher of water which I keep chilled in the fridge. The water tastes great, and it is pure, healthy, inexpensive, and does not contribute to pollution.

Do stay away from soda. It is full of high fructose corn syrup and artificial colors and flavors. If you think diet soda is better, t isn't. The artificial sweeteners in it are extremely unhealthy. When you are eating right and drinking enough water, cravings for soda tend to disappear. One thing I love to do is mix about one tablespoon of frozen juice concentrate such as orange or grape into a glass of water or sparkling water (with no additives). It gives the water flavor without adding too many calories or sugar. This is a great alternative to soda and commercial flavored drinks. It's much healthier and less expensive too.

Studies have shown that one alcoholic drink per day (especially of red wine) is good for health. I believe this is probably true. However, alcohol is also an addictive depressant and causes serious weight gain when over-used. If you have any trouble at all limiting yourself to one alcoholic beverage per day, I would recommend staying away from it all together.

Caffeine is an addictive stimulant and should also be limited. Coffee especially is not particularly good for your digestive tract because of its acidity. However, as with alcohol, it has been shown that one to two cups per day can have a healthy effect. So, if you aren't overly sensitive to the caffeine or the acidity, there is nothing wrong with consuming one or two cups per day (unless, of course, you are pregnant). If you do, please choose organic, free-trade coffee. Coffee crops tend to be highly contaminated with pesticides, and when you don't buy free-trade coffee, you support an industry that treats workers very poorly and does not pay fair value to plantation owners in the developing world.

The healthiest caffeinated drink is actually tea. Green tea especially is very mild in terms of caffeine content and has many health benefits such as high antioxidant content. The world of full-leaf fine tea is fascinating. One of the most enjoyable changes I've made in my life has been the switch from coffee to tea and subsequently learning about all the different varieties of tea.

Herbal infusions (commonly referred to as herbal teas) are wonderful, healthful beverages and definitely count towards your water intake since they are free of caffeine. Some fantastically healthy and delicious herbal infusions can be made from plants such as ginger, ginseng, chamomile, linden, anise, and more. I encourage you to try several herbal teas and drink them hot or cold. There is an infinite variety there just begging to be explored.

FOODS TO AVOID

I have mentioned many times so far that you should check labels and avoid unhealthy additives.

People often complain about the idea of reading ingredient labels as if by doing so they would be losing hours from their lives. It's really not that hard to just take a moment to look at an ingredient list before tossing something into your shopping cart. After all, you are planning on putting this food in your body and letting your family eat it too. Don't you think it would be wise to have some idea of what's in it? Once you learn what to look for and avoid, the whole process of reading labels becomes just another habit, and it's not a big deal.

Eliminate completely
- Meat, animal milk, eggs and all their byproducts
- High fructose corn syrup
- Anything hydrogenated or partially hydrogenated
- Casein or caseinate
- Whey
- Gelatin
- Artificial flavors
- Artificial colors (like Red #40 etc.)
- Anything that doesn't sound like food!

Limit intake of
- Sugar - Read the nutrition facts part of the label, and keep your daily grams of sugars as low as possible. It should definitely stay below 40 which is the equivalent of 10 teaspoons.
- Sodium - Read the nutrition facts part of labels, and do not buy anything that has a sodium content above 10% of the daily recommended amount in one serving.

Now that I've brought up sugar, I want to point out that as with other foods, the less processed the sugar the better. Buy unbleached, organic sugar whenever possible. My favorite brand is Florida Crystals. Do stay away completely from high fructose corn syrup. It is a substance made from corn starch treated with enzymes to convert glucose to fructose. It is hidden in all kinds of processed foods these days and has contributed to the rise of obesity in the United States. If the health effects of sugar worry you a lot, and you want to cut it out completely, try some of the natural sugar substitutes found in the health food store. These are much better for you than the artificial processed sweeteners so prevalent these days. Stevia, xylitol, and agave nectar are the most popular sugar substitutes, and they are healthy in moderation and all natural. Do note that stevia is much sweeter than sugar and requires only a fraction of the amount. Xylitol can be substituted one to one. Processed sugar in excessive amounts has been linked to weight gain, diabetes, tooth decay, mood swings, and a depressed immune system. These are excellent reasons to keep your daily intake below 40 grams.

Honestly, that is just a small start in the right direction. There are tons of things typically put into processed foods that are not wholesome and healthful. That is why the best way to avoid that stuff is to base your diet on whole foods. There are no labels on fruits and vegetables. Occasionally, though, we all want to go for the familiar or the convenient, so just be careful when you do.

Here is a simple comparison of two products that illustrates why reading labels is worthwhile. I used to love Kellogg's Pop Tarts. Even after cutting animal products out of my diet, I kept eating them because the unfrosted varieties are vegan. However, now that I am interested in eating healthfully, I would never eat one. Instead, when I crave a Pop Tart, I buy Nature's Path Toaster Pastries instead. They aren't exactly health food, but they are okay for an occasional treat, the ingredients are a lot better than those in Pop Tarts, and they taste better too. Now see for yourself:

Kellogg's Pop Tarts Unfrosted Strawberry
Strawberry Filling (Corn Syrup, Dextrose, High Fructose Corn Syrup, Crackermeal, Water, Modified Wheat Starch, Partially Hydrogenated Soybean Oil, Dried Strawberries, Dried Apples, Dried Pears, Citric Acid, Caramel Color, Red #40, Xanthan Gum, Soy Lecithin, Yellow #6), Enriched Wheat Flour, Partially Hydrogenated Soybean Oil, Corn Syrup, Sugar, Dextrose, Salt, High Fructose Corn Syrup, Leavening (Baking Soda, Sodium Acid Pyrophosphate, Monocalcium Phosphate), Niacinamide, Reduced Iron, Vitamin A Palmitate, Pyridoxine Hydrochloride (Vitamin B6), Riboflavin (Vitamin B2), Thiamin Hydrochloride (Vitamin B1), and Folic Acid.

Nature's Path Toaster Pastries Unfrosted Strawberry
Organic wheat flour, organic evaporated cane juice, organic palm oil, organic apples, organic whole wheat flour, organic corn starch, organic vital wheat gluten, organic dextrose, organic strawberries, organic rice starch, organic strawberry flavor, sea salt, leavening (baking soda, cream of tartar), organic rice bran extract, organic honey, organic molasses, citric acid, colored with betalains (from plants) & paprika extract, organic vanilla flavor.

I think that most people would agree that one of those lists is clearly more wholesome than the other. You don't need to be a nutritionist to tell. Every part of our bodies is all-natural and alive. Why would we want to consume synthetic, artificial substances? So, when faced with options, spend a moment comparing labels, and use a little common sense. It is really worth it. If you are not sure about what an ingredient is, look it up online. There is no excuse for anyone with internet access to say that they don't know what is in their food.

ABOUT VITAMINS

One of the joys of eating a balanced plant-based diet is that you are practically assured of getting enough of the vital nutrients that our bodies need. As long as you eat whole grains, beans, and a variety of colorful fruits and vegetables, you are going to do great in the nutrition department. In fact, meat eaters are far more likely in general to suffer from nutritional deficiencies than vegetarians are.

Eating the way I have described above will give you sufficient protein, calcium, fiber, and other vitamins and minerals.

There is one – just one – vitamin that those who eat a healthy plant-based diet are sometimes found to be deficient in. That is vitamin B12. That is the one vitamin that seems to occur abundantly only in animal-based foods. B12 is produced by bacteria that are only present in soil and on decomposing flesh. The only ways to obtain it through diet are to eat meat (which we've established you should not do), or to eat your vegetables raw and with soil on them (which for obvious reasons of sanitation you should not do). For this reason, I agree with the many expert opinions that those who eat only plant-based foods should use a B12 supplement or enough fortified foods to get your daily requirement. Some might try to use this fact as proof that a plant-based diet isn't optimum, but I disagree. Nothing is perfect in this world, and the many benefits to living on plant-based foods far outweigh the possible lack of this one vitamin as far as I and many experts are concerned.

To cover my B12 requirement I eat nutritional yeast often. I also take a look at the labels on my breakfast cereal and soy milk or almond milk to see how much B12 I'm getting that way. If you have any doubt, taking a multivitamin with B12 in it, or a dedicated B12 vitamin is a great thing to do. My vitamin

B12 levels have always been excellent whether I supplement or not, so I think the fortified foods and nutritional yeast really cover it. Plus, it is stored by the body for a LONG time, so it would take a long time of getting zero B12 to develop a deficiency.

Nutritional yeast tips

- Red Star brand, Bob's Red Mill brand, or in the Whole Foods bulk self-serve area
- Sprinkle it on pasta dishes, any and all cooked veggies, and popcorn. It is quite tasty, almost cheesy and a great vegan source of B12.

I also recommend that you eat ground flax seeds often for a good source of Omega 3's. Vitamin D supplementation is a good idea for almost everyone – vegan or not.

Please consult your doctor in terms of vitamin and mineral supplementation. Get tested for your levels and follow his or her advice. Obviously, when pregnant or lactating, please be extra vigilant about getting all the nutrients you need. I had a very successful vegan pregnancy and breast-feeding period. But, I did supplement a lot (like everyone should – vegan or not) and followed my doctor's advice to a T.

Planning meals

Now I want to give you some practical advice on what to eat on a daily basis. This basically summarizes the concepts I have presented so far and should help you to put it all into practice.

When you are eating the optimum diet I have been describing, you don't need to count calories, or limit your intake. All you have to do is make sure that you eat a great variety of the foods I've discussed. Be adventurous, try different things, and above all keep yourself satisfied. I've heard people complain that they tried to be vegetarian, but they were hungry all the time and couldn't keep it up. Well, I'll show you here that there is no reason to ever feel hungry.

One important thing I've learned is that it is best to eat many times throughout the day to avoid peaks and valleys in your energy level. Don't let yourself get hungry to the point where you gorge yourself. I have found that I need to eat something every 3 hours or so, even if it is just a small handful of nuts or dried fruit.

Breakfast

Start the day off right with whole grains and some good fat. These foods will give you long-lasting energy. Avoid sugar and refined flour at breakfast time. Good options are:

- A fruit smoothie and a piece of whole wheat toast with almond butter or peanut butter
- A bowl of whole grain hot cereal (like oatmeal) with a little soymilk, maple syrup, chopped nuts, and bananas or berries
- Nondairy yogurt with granola and berries
- Cold whole grain cereal with almond milk and a banana
- Pancakes made with whole wheat flour and fruit
- Scrambled tofu and whole grain toast

Lunch

I find the best lunch options to be salad or leftovers from the previous night's dinner. I love having containers of prewashed salad greens and precut veggies in the fridge to make lunch an easy matter to put together. Here are some ideas:

- Reheated leftovers from dinner
- A salad with a flax oil vinaigrette that includes some beans (like chickpeas or kidney beans) and some nuts (like chopped walnuts or slivered almonds)
- A wrap or sandwich with hummus or avocado and any fresh vegetables you like
- A sandwich made with Tofurkey deli slices and salad greens
- A wrap with black beans, avocado, and salsa
- A PB&J sandwich with carrots and celery on the side

Snacks

I eat all day long (and no, I'm not overweight). There is a multitude of foods you can eat when hunger strikes between meals. I highly recommend having your favorite snack foods handy at all times. Keep food at home, at your office, and in your bag that you carry all day. Being stuck where there are no good food choices and feeling ravenously hungry is a bad situation to be in. My favorite snack foods are:

- Cut up fresh veggies (carrots, celery, bell peppers, etc.)
- A piece of fruit (especially apples, bananas, and oranges)
- Nondairy yogurt with or without a little granola
- A handful of nuts and/or seeds
- A handful of dried fruit
- A piece of toast or crackers with almond butter or peanut butter
- A fruit smoothie
- A whole food snack bar like a Larabar or Clif Nectar bar

Dinner

For dinner, I can't stress enough the value of planning your meals in advance. I do my menu planning and shopping once a week so I know that I have everything I need to make dinner every night. This ensures that I make a wide variety of dishes so that nothing gets boring and so that all the nutritional bases get covered throughout the week. I also rarely make anything that requires more than 30 minutes to put together. If you tend to have very little time to put a meal together in the evening, try to do as much preparation the night before or in the morning. You can chop up the veggies, and put them in ziplock bags. You can precook your grain and reheat it at dinner time. Again, plan ahead! These are habits that may take some effort to develop, but I'm sure you can figure out a way to structure your time so that you can be sure to eat properly. You have to get your priorities straight!

Check out the many vegan cookbooks and resources online, but also remember that there are many things you already eat that can easily be made healthier and vegan. I personally love to alter traditional recipes. It's also great fun to make foods from different ethnic cuisines. I make dishes from all over Asia, from India, from Latin America, etc. I never used to like cooking, but now that I am on a mission to eat healthfully, cooking has become a pleasure. I love knowing exactly what goes into the food I eat, and I love the feeling of satisfaction I get from knowing that I am not dependent on restaurants and takeout. So, at dinner time, be creative, learn new recipes, be open-minded, and enjoy yourself.

Most dinners should include vegetables, a grain, and some protein in the form of beans, tofu, seitan, tempeh, or the occasional commercial meat substitute.

Dessert

I don't know about you, but I can't live without dessert. Dinner is just not complete for me without something sweet to finish it off. This is also the time when I indulge in foods that you might not exactly call healthy. Because I avoid sugar and refined flour at all other times, I let myself have them in moderation at dessert time.

Here are some of my favorite after-dinner treats:

- A piece of dairy-free organic dark chocolate (read the label)
- A scoop of non-dairy ice cream
- A scoop of sorbet
- A couple of vegan cookies (Whole Foods brand makes several)
- Non-dairy yogurt
- Fruit
- Any of the many delicious baked goods you can learn to make

TABLES AND LISTS

Here I'm going to reiterate in simple list form the basic information about what foods to eat and what things to avoid. Refer to this section often, especially when making a shopping list!

Eat in abundance

Grains

- Brown rice
- Quinoa
- Bulgur wheat
- Barley
- Millet
- Oatmeal
- Whole grain pasta

Vegetables

- Dark leafy greens (kale, chard, organic spinach...)
- Onions
- Garlic
- Ginger
- Carrots
- Bell peppers (organic)
- Shiitake mushrooms
- Tomatoes
- Sweet potatoes
- Beets
- Broccoli
- Sea vegetables (dulse, kelp, nori, wakame)

Fruits

- Oranges
- Bananas
- Blueberries

- Other berries
- Apples (organic)

Nuts and seeds

- Macadamias
- Hazelnuts
- Pecans
- Almonds
- Walnuts
- Cashews
- Ground flax seeds
- Sesame seeds
- Pumpkin seeds
- Almond butter
- Cashew butter
- Peanut butter (organic, no salt or sugar added)

Proteins

- Tofu (organic)
- Tempeh (organic)
- Seitan
- Beans of any kind
- Occasional commercial mock meat

Oils (in moderation)

- Extra-virgin olive oil
- Canola oil
- Peanut oil
- Flaxseed oil (drizzle cold oil on prepared food)

Eliminate

- Meat, animal milk, and eggs
- Casein or caseinate
- Whey
- High fructose corn syrup

- Anything hydrogenated or partially hydrogenated
- Gelatin
- Artificial flavors
- Artificial colors (like Red #40 etc.)

Limit

- Any ingredient you don't recognize
- Sugar - read nutrition facts to stay under 40 grams per day)
- Sodium - don't let any one item contain more than 10% of the daily limit)

When to choose organic

- Bell peppers
- Dark green leafies
- Potatoes
- Celery
- Corn
- Lettuces
- Peaches
- Apples
- Nectarines
- Strawberries
- Cherries
- Pears
- Grapes
- Raisins
- Soy products
- Peanuts
- Coffee
- Chocolate

The best meat substitutes

Meat Product	Vegetarian Substitute
Raw Ground Beef	Lightlife Gimme Lean Ground Beef Style
Browned Ground Beef	Lightlife Smart Ground WestSoy Ground seitan Tofurky ground beef style
Beef Strips or Chunks	Lightlife Steak Style Strips Gardein Homestyle Beefless Tips (frozen) WestSoy Seitan
Beef Burgers	Amy's All American Burger (frozen) Boca Original Vegan (frozen) Make from scratch with Gimme Lean
Meatballs	Nate's (frozen) Whole Foods (frozen) Make meatballs with Lightlife Gimme Lean
Chicken Patties or Cutlets	Gardein Chick'n Scalloppini (frozen) Boca Original Chik'n Patties (frozen)
Chicken Strips or Chunks	Lightlife Chick'n Strips Beyond Meat Chicken Free Strips Gardein Chick'n Scalloppini (frozen)
Hot Dogs	Lightlife Tofu Pups
Breakfast Sausage	Field Roast Apple Sage or Apple Maple
Italian Sausage	Lightlife Gimme Lean Sausage Style (crumbled) Tofurkey Artisan line Field Roast Grain Meat Sausages - Italian
Other sausage	Field Roast Smoked Apple Sage Sausage Field Roast Mexican Tofurkey Artisan Spinach Pesto
Bacon	Lightlife Smart Bacon Lightlife Fakin' Bacon tempeh

Deli Meats	Field Roast Deli Slices Tofurkey Deli Slices
Meatloaf	Field Roast Classic Meatloaf Make from Scratch with Gimme Lean
Roasted Turkey	Field Roast Celebration Roast Tofurkey Roast (frozen)

The best dairy substitutes

Dairy Product	Dairy-Free Substitute
Butter	Earth Balance Buttery Spread
Milk	Whole Foods Brand WestSoy Almond Breeze Dream Blends (highly fortified. Best for kids!) So Delicious
Yogurt	So Delicious Cultured Coconut Milk Almond Dream Yogurt WholeSoy Yogurt
Cream Cheese	Tofutti Better Than Cream Cheese * Get the "Non Hydrogenated Plain"
Sour Cream	Tofutti Better than Sour Cream
Ice Cream	So Delicious (almond, soy, or coconut based)
Cream	Silk Original Creamer So Delicious
Whipped Cream	Soyatoo Soy Whip
Parmesan Cheese	Galaxy Foods Vegan Grated Topping
Mayonnaise	Vegenaise Nayonaise (more like Miracle Whip)

The best miscellaneous products

- Many Whole Foods brand products
- Vermont Bread Company sandwich bread
- Cascadian Farm cereals
- Kashi breakfast cereals
- Frozen fruit and vegetables from Whole Foods brand, Cascadian Farm, or Earthbound
- Arrowhead Mills and Bob's Red Mill hot cereals, grains, and baking ingredients like flour, baking powder and soda, cornstarch, etc.
- Arrowhead Mills nut butters
- Florida Crystals sugar
- Larabar snack bars
- Clif Nectar snack bars

Vitamins

Check on your B12 intake (use nutritional yeast and fortified foods), and follow your doctor's advice on vitamin supplementation. Most people need D supplements whether they are vegan or not!

Eat ground flax seeds for your Omega 3's (one tablespoon per day blended into your smoothie, mixed with yogurt, or sprinkled on cereal or veggies)

Recipe substitutions

For eggs in baked goods

- use Ener-G or Bob's Red Mill powdered egg replacer. Or...
- For each egg in your recipe, combine 1 tablespoon ground flaxseeds with 2 tablespoons hot water. Allow to sit for about 3 minutes. Then whisk briskly.

For milk

- Use plain, unsweetened soymilk or almond milk

For butter

- Use Earth Balance in equal measure

FREQUENTLY ASKED QUESTIONS

You probably still have some questions about all of this. Hopefully, I will address most of them here, and the answers will dispel any lingering doubts you might have and will be useful to you when people in your life inevitably start asking you about your new habits.

Where do you get your protein?

This is one of the most common questions vegetarians get asked. I find it quite funny because people who don't seem to give a hoot about their own health and nutrition suddenly become experts on protein deficiency if anyone tells them they are a vegan. You should know by now that the answer to this is that there is absolutely no proof that vegetarians or vegans tend to suffer from protein deficiency. On the contrary, meat eaters tend to get too much protein which leads to calcium loss and other ill effects. Beans, nuts, and grains contain plenty of healthy protein.

Where do you get your calcium?

This is another common one. The answer is that calcium is a mineral that comes from plants. The only reason it is even in cow's milk is because the cows traditionally got it from grass, though now that dairy cows are rarely fed grass, they actually just get it in supplement form. Dark green vegetables contain all the calcium humans need. Since consuming animal protein actually draws calcium out of the body, vegetarians do better in the calcium department than people who consume dairy products and meat.

Aren't humans natural carnivores?

No. We are omnivores. That means we technically can eat just about anything. However, we are much more suited to a vegetarian diet and thrive on it. In a way, though, I feel that the question isn't even relevant. We've clearly evolved as a species to do things our ancestors never imagined themselves capable of doing. I think that in this modern world in which there are so many food choices and so much knowledge, it makes more sense to be a vegetarian than to breed and kill animals in unprecedented numbers just to satisfy our desire to eat them. So many studies show that people who live on a varied plant-based diet are healthier and live longer than people who don't.

Milk is bad for you?

The animal agriculture business has awesome economic and political power. They have the money and the incentive to bombard you constantly with false claims that their products are good for you. Do not take their word for it. Educate yourself. They even have the government producing ads for them. Have you ever seen the ads for cheese that say "Great cheese comes from happy cows. Happy cows come from California"? Those ads are a gross example of false advertising because, of course, the cows are anything but happy. However, because the ads are produced by a government agency, they are exempt from false advertising laws. Multiple law suits against these ads have failed in court not because they aren't making false claims but because they are produced by the California Milk Board and not a corporate entity.

Isn't too much soy bad for you?

There has been some concern about whether soy products might actually be harmful. However, there is far more conclusive evidence that soy is beneficial than that it causes harm. There has been no proof that soy is anything but healthy. I'd like to say, however, that the very healthiest soy products are the whole, organic ones: organic fresh soybeans (edamame), organic tofu, and organic tempeh. When a food is highly processed, there is always the possibility that its health benefits can be compromised. That seems to be the situation with soy. There's also the fact that no one food should be eaten in excess. That is why throughout this book I've stressed the importance of a varied, whole-foods diet. Take it easy on the processed soy-based meat substitutes, and use almond milk or rice milk for variety.

Isn't it hard to be a strict vegan?
No. It really is not difficult. At first, there is a learning curve, and you have to establish new habits. Once you are used to eating right, though, it's just as easy as eating poorly. You just get to a point where you know what's good for you and what you like, you know where to shop, you know what to buy, and you learn to always have good food on hand. If you do it right, eating a wholesome plant-based diet is a very simple matter.

Isn't it expensive?
No. Beans, seitan, and tofu are much cheaper than meat. Anyway, the only reason meat is so cheap is because it is subsidized by the government with our tax money. Good produce can also be had inexpensively, especially if you buy in season. Even better, you should try to buy local produce at farmer's markets. What tend to be expensive are the imitation meats, dairy substitutes, and sometimes organic produce. That's another good reason to stick to whole foods rather than processed ones. Remember too, that if need be you can go with regular produce, especially if it's not on my list called "When to go organic". Also even if you did spend more on a healthy diet (which you probably won't), the chances are good that you will save on medical costs in the long run because a healthy diet helps prevent disease.

What do you do when you eat out?
A lot of people go vegan at home first before extending it to their activities out in the world. (Or go vegan at home and lacto-ovo vegetarian when out.) I think this is a perfectly fine

approach when you are starting out. What I think will happen (and what happened to me) is that as you get more used to eating vegan most of the time, you will really want to start doing it outside your home as well and you will just do it!

When it comes to eating out, your habits will probably have to change a bit. Here are some tips: Asian and Indian restaurants tend to be very vegan friendly. They usually have several choices on the menu and are also happy to alter a dish for you. I will often request tofu instead of shrimp or chicken in a stir fry and ask for the egg to be omitted from my fried rice, for example. It hasn't ever been a problem. At Italian restaurants, you can ask for a pizza with no cheese or pasta with olive oil or marinara sauce and no cheese. At Mexican restaurants, too, it is easy to request a dish with no meat or cheese – beans, vegetables, and salsa are perfectly sufficient. In short, get to know the kinds of restaurants that are easiest to eat at, and don't be afraid to make special requests.

I found some great web pages with advice on how to eat vegan at chain restaurants. Check *veganfirststeps.com* for up-to-date links. Even if you don't eat at these types of places, the tips can help guide you in how to look at menus and figure out what to eat. As I mentioned before, most places will happily piece something together for you if you are clear about what you want!

Is this a weight-loss diet?

No, it's not. However, if you are currently overweight and change your habits to match what I have described in this book, there is a very good chance that you will lose weight and keep it off. Because a varied plant-based diet is naturally high in fiber and low in fat and calories, most people who live this lifestyle stay at a healthy weight for them. If you are particularly concerned with losing weight, it is best to make fresh fruits and vegetables the bulk of your food intake, and eat grains, nuts, seeds, and proteins moderately by comparison. Also, be especially careful of sugar and refined flour. You may want to stick to fruit for dessert until you are at a healthy weight. Don't forget that no matter how you eat, exercise is very important for maintaining a healthy weight too.

What's a vegan?

A person who identifies himself or herself as a vegan believes that animals should not be used as commodities for humans in any way. Not only do they not eat animals and products made by and from animals, but they also buy only animal-free clothing and do not use personal care products that were tested on animals, for example. If you follow the eating guidelines in this book to the letter, you will essentially be eating the same way as a vegan. However, you are not technically a vegan unless your primary reason for following that regimen is the rights of animals, and to be a true vegan you must go further than just changing your eating habits.

How do I deal with friends and family?

With friends, I suggest saying that you have been trying eating a vegan diet to see what it feels like, and ask if they would they mind humoring you. Be aware that people tend to feel judged when someone says they don't eat meat, so ease your friends and family into it.

Do I have to go vegan overnight?

I am not what I'd call a "militant" type of vegan. I'm all for helping people make incremental changes. However, some people can't really do things unless they do them all the way. So, you will be the best judge of how far you should try to go with it right off the bat and how abruptly. I know that I feel great as a 100% vegan (even in my clothing and household products), and I knew it was the only way I could raise my son.

But any steps you take towards veganism will change your life for the better, I believe.

Where do I get more information?

My website is at *veganfirststeps.com*. I will maintain a list of resources there.